MW01264795

# Renal Diet Everyday Recipes

A Complete Renal Diet Cookbook to Prepare Recipes for Those on Dialysis with Low Sodium, Low Potassium, and Low Phosphorus

## Vanessa Hayes

© Copyright 2021 – Vanessa Hayes - All rights
reserved.

The content contained within this book may not be
reproduced, duplicated or transmitted without direct written
permission from the author or the publisher.
Under no circumstances will any blame or legal responsibility
be held against the publisher, or author, for any damages,
reparation, or monetary loss due to the information contained
within this book. Either directly or indirectly.

**Legal Notice:**

This book is copyright protected. This book is only for
personal use. You cannot amend, distribute, sell, use, quote or
paraphrase any part, or the content within this book, without
the consent of the author or publisher.

**Disclaimer Notice:**

Please note the information contained within this document is
for educational and entertainment purposes only. All effort
has been executed to present accurate, up to date, and reliable,
complete information. No warranties of any kind are declared
or implied. Readers acknowledge that the author is not

engaging in the rendering of legal, financial, medical or professional advice. The content within this book has been derived from various sources. Please consult a licensed professional before attempting any techniques outlined in this book.

By reading this document, the reader agrees that under no circumstances is the author responsible for any losses, direct or indirect, which are incurred as a result of the use of information contained within this document, including, but not limited to, errors, omissions, or inaccuracies.

# Table of Content

# Breakfast

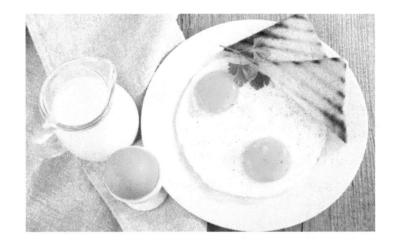

# Carrot Jicama Salad

Preparation Time: 5 minutes

Cooking Time: 0 minutes

Servings: 2

Ingredients:

- 2 cup carrots, julienned
- 1 1/2 cups jicama, julienned
- 2 tablespoons lime juice
- 1 tablespoon olive oil
- ½ tablespoon apple cider
- ½ teaspoon brown Swerve

Direction:

1. Put all the salad ingredients into a suitable salad bowl.
2. Toss them well and refrigerate for 1 hour.
3. Serve.

Nutrition: Calories 173 Total Fat 7.1g Sodium 80mg Protein 1.6g Calcium 50mg Phosphorous 96mg Potassium 501mg

# Salmon and Carrots Mix

Preparation Time: 10 minutes

Cooking Time: 10 minutes

Servings: 4

Ingredients:

- 4 oz. chopped smoked salmon
- 1 tbsp. essential olive oil
- Black pepper
- 1 tbsp. chopped chives
- ¼ c. coconut cream
- 1 ½ lbs. chopped carrots
- 2 tsps. Prepared horseradish

Directions:

1. Heat up a pan using the oil over medium heat, add carrots and cook for 10 minutes.

2. Add salmon, chives, horseradish, cream and black pepper, toss, cook for 1 minute more, divide between plates and serve.

3. Enjoy!

Nutrition: Calories: 233, Fat: 6 g, Carbs: 9 g, Protein: 11 g, Sugars: 3.3 g, Sodium: 97 mg

# Baked Fennel & Garlic Sea Bass

Preparation Time: 5 minutes

Cooking Time: 15 minutes

Servings: 2

Ingredients:

- 1 lemon
- ½ sliced fennel bulb
- 6 oz. sea bass fillets
- 1 tsp black pepper
- 2 garlic cloves

Directions:

1.    Preheat the oven to 375°F. Sprinkle black pepper over the Sea Bass. Slice the fennel bulb and garlic cloves. Add 1 salmon fillet and half the fennel and garlic to one sheet of baking paper or tin foil.

2.    Squeeze in 1/2 lemon juices. Repeat for the other fillet. Fold and add to the oven for 12-15 minutes or until fish is thoroughly cooked through.

3.    Meanwhile, add boiling water to your couscous, cover, and allow to steam. Serve with your choice of rice or salad.

Nutrition: Calories 221 Protein 14 g Carbs 3 g Fat 2 g Sodium 119 mg Potassium 398 mg Phosphorus 149 mg

# Shrimp Lo Mein

Preparation Time: 10 minutes

Cooking Time: 10 minutes

Servings: 6

Ingredients:

- 1 tbsp. cornstarch
- 1 lb. medium-size frozen raw shrimp
- 1 c. frozen shelled edamame
- 3 tbsps. Light teriyaki sauce
- 16 oz. Drained and rinsed tofu spaghetti noodles
- 18 oz. frozen Szechuan vegetable blend with sesame sauce

Directions:

1. Microwave noodles for 1 minute; set aside. Place shrimp in a small bowl and toss with 2 tablespoons teriyaki sauce; set aside.

2. Place mixed vegetables and edamame in a large nonstick skillet with 1/4 cup water. Cover and cook, stirring occasionally, over medium-high heat for 7 minutes or until cooked through.

3. Stir shrimp into vegetable mixture; cover and cook 4 to 5 minutes or until shrimp is pink and cooked through.

4. Stir together remaining 1 tablespoon teriyaki sauce and the cornstarch, then stir into the mixture in the skillet until

thickened. Gently stir noodles into skillet and cook until warmed through.

Nutrition: Calories: 252, Fat: 7.1 g, Carbs: 35.2 g, Protein: 12.1 g, Sugars: 2.2 g, Sodium: 180 mg

# Sardine Fish Cakes

Preparation Time: 10 minutes

Cooking Time: 10 minutes

Servings: 4

Ingredients:

- 11 oz. sardines, canned, drained
- 1/3 cup shallot, chopped
- 1 teaspoon chili flakes
- ½ teaspoon salt
- 2 tablespoon wheat flour, whole grain
- 1 egg, beaten
- 1 tablespoon chives, chopped
- 1 teaspoon olive oil
- 1 teaspoon butter

Directions:

1.     Put the butter in your skillet and dissolve it. Add shallot and cook it until translucent. After this, transfer the shallot to the mixing bowl.

2.     Add sardines, chili flakes, salt, flour, egg, chives, and mix up until smooth with the fork's help.   Make the medium size cakes and place them in the skillet. Add olive oil.

3.     Roast the fish cakes for 3 minutes from each side over medium heat. Dry the cooked fish cakes with a paper towel if needed and transfer to the serving plates.

Nutrition: Calories 221 Fat 12.2g Fiber 0.1g Carbs 5.4g Protein 21.3 g  Phosphorus 188.7 mg Potassium 160.3 mg Sodium 452.6 mg

# Cod and Green Bean Curry

Preparation Time: 15 min

Cooking Time: 60 minutes

Servings: 4

Ingredients:

- 1/2-pound green beans, trimmed and cut into bite-sized pieces
- 1 white onion, sliced
- 2 cloves garlic, minced
- 1 tablespoon olive oil, or more as needed
- Ground black pepper to taste
- Curry Mixture:
- 2 tablespoons water, or more as needed
- 2 teaspoons curry powder
- 2 teaspoons ground ginger
- 1 1/2 (6 ounce) cod fillets

Directions:

1. Preheat the oven to 400 degrees F.

2. Combine green beans, onion, and garlic in a large glass baking dish. Toss with olive oil to coat; season with the pepper.

3. Bake in the preheated oven, stirring occasionally, until edges of onion are slightly charred and green beans start to look dry, about 40 minutes. In the meantime, mix water, curry powder, and ginger together.

4.     Remove dish and stir the vegetables; stir in curry mixture. Increase oven temperature to 450 degrees F.

5.     Lay cod over the bottom of the dish and coat with vegetables. Continue baking until fish is opaque, 25 to 30 minutes depending on thickness.

Nutrition: Calories 64, Total Fat 3.8g, Saturated Fat 0.5g, Cholesterol 0mg, Sodium 5mg, Total Carbohydrate 7.7g, Dietary Fiber 2.9g, Total Sugars 2g, Protein 1.6g, Calcium 35mg, Iron 1mg, Potassium 180mg, Phosphorus 101 mg

# Cranberry Cabbage Slaw

Preparation Time: 5 minutes

Cooking Time: 0 minutes

Servings: 4

Ingredients:

- 1/2 medium cabbage head, shredded
- 1 medium red apple, shredded
- 2 tablespoons onion, sliced
- 1/2 cup dried cranberries
- 1/4 cup almonds, toasted sliced
- 1/2 cup olive oil
- ¼ teaspoon stevia
- 1/4 cup cider vinegar
- 1/2 tablespoon celery seed
- 1/2 teaspoon dry mustard
- ½ cup cream

Direction:

1. Take a suitable salad bowl.

2. Start tossing in all the ingredients.

3. Mix well and serve.

Nutrition: Calories 308 Total Fat 24.5g Sodium 23mg Protein 2.6g Calcium 69mg Phosphorous 257mg Potassium 219mg

# Cod & Green Bean Risotto

Preparation Time: 4 minutes

Cooking Time: 40 minutes

Servings: 2

Ingredients:

- ½ cup arugula
- 1 finely diced white onion
- 4 oz. cod fillet
- 1 cup white rice
- 2 lemon wedges
- 1 cup boiling water
- ¼ tsp. black pepper
- 1 cup low-sodium chicken broth
- 1 tbsp. extra virgin olive oil
- ½ cup green beans

Directions:

1. Warm-up oil in a large pan on medium heat. Sauté the chopped onion for 5 minutes until soft before adding in the rice and stirring for 1-2 minutes.

2. Combine the broth with boiling water. Add half of the liquid to the pan and stir. Slowly add the rest of the liquid while continuously stirring for up to 20-30 minutes.

3. Stir in the green beans to the risotto. Place the fish on top of the rice, cover, and steam for 10 minutes.

4. Use your fork to break up the fish fillets and stir into the rice. Sprinkle with freshly ground pepper to serve and a

squeeze of fresh lemon. Serve with the lemon wedges and the arugula.

Nutrition: Calories 221 Protein 12 g Carbs 29 g Fat 8 g Sodium 398 mg Potassium 347 mg Phosphorus 241 mg

# Lemon, Garlic, Cilantro Tuna and Rice

Preparation Time: 5 minutes

Cooking Time: 0 minutes

Servings: 2

Ingredients:

- ½ cup arugula
- 1 tbsp. extra virgin olive oil
- 1 cup cooked rice
- 1 tsp black pepper
- ¼ finely diced red onion
- 1 juiced lemon
- 3 oz. canned tuna
- 2 tbsp. Chopped fresh cilantro

Directions:

1.    Mix the olive oil, pepper, cilantro, and red onion in a bowl. Stir in the tuna, cover, then serve with the cooked rice and arugula!

Nutrition: Calories 221 Protein 11 g Carbs 26 g Fat 7 g Sodium 143 mg Potassium 197 mg Phosphorus 182 mg

# Easy Salmon and Brussels sprouts

Preparation Time: 10 minutes

Cooking Time: 10 minutes

Servings: 6


Ingredients:

- 6 deboned medium salmon fillets
- 1 tsp. onion powder
- 1 ¼ lbs. halved Brussels sprouts
- 3 tbsps. Extra virgin extra virgin olive oil
- 2 tbsps. Brown sugar
- 1 tsp. garlic powder
- 1 tsp. smoked paprika


Directions:

1. In a bowl, mix sugar with onion powder, garlic powder, smoked paprika as well as a number of tablespoon olive oil and whisk well.

2. Spread Brussels sprouts about the lined baking sheet, drizzle the rest in the essential extra virgin olive oil, toss to coat, introduce in the oven at 450 0F and bake for 5 minutes.

3. Add salmon fillets brush with sugar mix you've prepared, introduce inside the oven and bake for 15 minutes more.

4. Divide everything between plates and serve.

5.     Enjoy!

Nutrition: Calories: 212, Fat: 5 g, Carbs: 12 g, Protein: 8 g, Sugars: 3.7 g, Sodium: 299.1 mg

# Butterscotch Apple Salad

Preparation Time: 5 minutes

Cooking Time: 0 minutes

Servings: 6

Ingredients:

- 3 cups jazz apples, chopped
- 8 oz. canned crushed pineapple
- 8 oz. whipped topping
- 1/2 cup butterscotch topping
- 1/3 cup almonds
- 1/4 cup butterscotch

Direction:

1. Put all the salad ingredients into a suitable salad bowl.
2. Toss them well and refrigerate for 1 hour.
3. Serve.

Nutrition: Calories 293 Total Fat 12.7g Sodium 52mg Protein 4.2g Calcium 65mg Phosphorous 202mg Potassium 296mg

# Steakhouse Soup

Preparation Time: 15 minutes

Cooking Time: 25 minutes

Servings: 4

Ingredients:

- 2 tbsps. soy sauce
- 2 boneless and cubed chicken breasts.
- ¼ lb. halved and trimmed snow peas
- 1 tbsp. minced ginger root
- 1 minced garlic clove
- 1 cup water
- 2 chopped green onions
- 3 cups chicken stock
- 1 chopped carrot
- 3 sliced mushrooms

Directions:

1.      Take a pot and combine ginger, water, chicken stock, Soy sauce (reduced salt) and garlic in this pot. Let them boil on medium heat, mix in chicken pieces, and let them simmer on low heat for almost 15 minutes to tender chicken.

2.      Stir in carrot and snow peas and simmer for almost 5 minutes. Add mushrooms in this blend and continue cooking to tender vegetables for nearly 3 minutes. Mix in the chopped onion and serve hot.

Nutrition: Calories 319, Carbs 14g, Fat 15g, Potassium (K) 225 mg, Protein 29g, Sodium (Na) 389 mg, Phosphorous 190 mg

# Onion Soup

Preparation Time: 15 minutes

Cooking Time: 45 minutes

Servings: 6

Ingredients:

- 2 tbsps. chicken stock
- 1 cup chopped Shiitake mushrooms
- 1 tbsp. minced chives
- 3 tsps. beef bouillon
- 1 tsp. grated ginger root
- ½ chopped carrot
- 1 cup sliced Portobello mushrooms
- 1 chopped onion
- ½ chopped celery stalk
- 2 quarts' water
- ¼ tsp. minced garlic

Directions:

1. Take a saucepan and combine carrot, onion, celery, garlic, mushrooms (some mushrooms) and ginger in this pan. Add water, beef bouillon and chicken stock in this pan. Put this pot on high heat and let it boil. Decrease flame to medium and cover this pan to cook for almost 45 minutes.

2. Put all remaining mushrooms in one separate pot. Once the boiling mixture is completely done, put one strainer over this new bowl with mushrooms and strain cooked soup in this pot over mushrooms. Discard solid-strained materials.

3.	Serve delicious broth with yummy mushrooms in small bowls and sprinkle chives over each bowl.

Nutrition: Calories 22, Fat 0g, Sodium (Na) 602.3mg, Potassium (K) 54.1mg, Carbs 4.9g, Protein 0.6g, Phosphorus 15.8mg

# Salmon in Dill Sauce

Preparation Time: 10 minutes

Cooking Time: 10 minutes

Servings: 6

Ingredients:

- 6 salmon fillets
- 1 c. low-fat, low-sodium chicken broth
- 1 tsp. cayenne pepper
- 2 tbsps. Fresh lemon juice
- 2 c. water
- ¼ c. chopped fresh dill

Directions:

1. In a slow cooker, mix together water, broth, lemon juice, lemon juice and dill.

2. Arrange salmon fillets on top, skin side down.

3. Sprinkle with cayenne pepper.

4. Set the slow cooker on low.

5. Cover and cook for about 1-2 hours.

Nutrition: Calories: 360, Fat: 8 g, Carbs: 44 g, Protein: 28 g, Sugars: 0.5 g, Sodium: 8 mg

# Tofu Soup

Preparation Time: 5 minutes

Cooking Time: 10 minutes

Servings: 2

Ingredients:

- 1 tbsp. miso paste
- 1/8 cup cubed soft tofu
- 1 chopped green onion
- ¼ cup sliced Shiitake mushrooms
- 3 cups Renali stock
- 1 tbsp. soy sauce

Directions:

1. Take a saucepan, pour the stock into this pan and let it boil on high heat. Reduce heat to medium and let this stock simmer. Add mushrooms in this stock and cook for almost 3 minutes.

2. Take a bowl and mix Soy sauce (reduced salt) and miso paste together in this bowl. Add this mixture and tofu in stock. Simmer for nearly 5 minutes and serve with chopped green onion.

Nutrition: Calories 129, Fat 7.8g, Sodium (Na) 484mg, Potassium (K) 435mg,Protein 11g, Carbs 5.5g, Phosphorus 73.2mg

# Grilled Cod

Preparation Time: 10 min

Cooking Time: 10 minutes

Servings: 4

Ingredients:

- 2 (8 ounce) fillets cod, cut in half
- 1 tablespoon oregano
- ½ teaspoon lemon pepper
- ¼ teaspoon ground black pepper
- 2 tablespoons olive oil
- 1 lemon, juiced
- 2 tablespoons chopped green onion (white part only)

Directions:

1.      Season both sides of cod with oregano, lemon pepper, and black pepper. Set fish aside on a plate. Heat butter in a small saucepan over medium heat, stir in lemon juice and green onion, and cook until onion is softened, about 3 minutes.

2.      Place cod onto oiled grates and grill until fish is browned and flakes easily, about 3 minutes per side; baste with olive oil mixture frequently while grilling. Allow cod to rest off the heat for about 5 minutes before serving.

Nutrition: Calories 92, Total Fat 7.4g, Saturated Fat 1g, Cholesterol 14mg, Sodium 19mg, Total Carbohydrate 2.5g, Dietary Fiber 1g, Total Sugars 0.5g, Protein 5.4g, Calcium 25mg, Iron 1mg, Potassium 50mg, Phosphorus 36 mg

# Stuffed Mushrooms

Preparation Time: 10 min

Cooking Time: 10 minutes

Servings: 4

Ingredients:

- 12 large fresh mushrooms, stems removed
- ½ pound crabmeat, flaked
- 2 cups olive oil
- 2 cloves garlic, peeled and minced
- Garlic powder to taste
- Crushed red pepper to taste

Directions:

1. Arrange mushroom caps on a medium baking sheet, bottoms up. Chop and reserve mushroom stems.

2. Preheat oven to 350 degrees F.

3. In a medium saucepan over medium heat, heat oil. Mix in garlic and cook until tender, about 5 minutes.

4. In a medium bowl, mix together reserved mushroom stems, and crab meat. Liberally stuff mushrooms with the mixture. Drizzle with the garlic. Season with garlic powder and crushed red pepper.

5. Bake uncovered in the preheated oven 10 to 12 minutes, or until stuffing is lightly browned.

Nutrition: Calories 312, Total Fat 33.8g, Saturated Fat 4.8g, Cholesterol 4mg, Sodium 160mg, Total Carbohydrate 3.8g,

Dietary Fiber 0.3g, Total Sugars 1.6g, Protein 2.2g, Calcium 3mg, Iron 1mg, Potassium 93mg, Phosphorus 86 mg

# Lunch

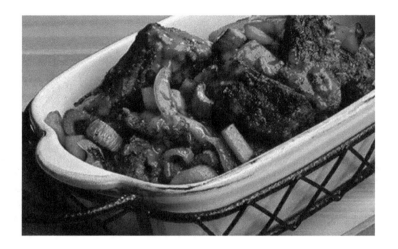

# Vegetable Rice Casserole

Preparation Time: 10 minutes

Cooking Time: 50 minutes

Servings: 4

Ingredients:

- 1 teaspoon of olive oil
- ½ small sweet onion, chopped
- ½ teaspoon of minced garlic
- ½ cup of chopped red bell pepper
- ¼ cup of grated carrot
- 1 cup of white basmati rice
- 2 cups of water
- ¼ cup of grated Parmesan cheese
- Freshly ground black pepper

Directions:

1. Preheat the oven to 350°f.

2. In a medium skillet over medium-high heat, heat the olive oil.

3. Add the onion and garlic, and sauté until softened, about 3 minutes.

4. Transfer the vegetables to a 9-by-9-inch baking dish, and stir in the rice and water.

5. Cover the dish and bake until the liquid is absorbed 35 to 40 minutes.

6. Sprinkle the cheese on top and bake an additional 5 minutes to melt.

7.     Season the casserole with pepper, and serve.

8.     Substitution tip: Not surprisingly, the cheesy topping on this casserole elevates it to a truly sublime experience. You can also try feta, Cheddar cheese, and goat cheese for different tastes and textures.

Nutrition: Calories: 224 Total fat: 3g Saturated fat: 1g Cholesterol: 6mg Sodium: 105mg Carbohydrates: 41g Fiber: 2g Phosphorus: 118mg Potassium: 176mg Protein: 6g

# Marinated Tofu Stir-Fry

Preparation time: 20 minutes

Cooking time: 20 minutes

Servings: 4 servings

Ingredients:

- For the tofu:
- Lemon juice – 1 tbsp.
- Minced garlic – 1 tsp
- Grated fresh ginger – 1 tsp
- Pinch red pepper flakes
- Extra-firm tofu- 5 ounces, pressed well and cubed
- For the stir-fry:
- Olive oil – 1 tbsp.
- Cauliflower florets – ½ cup
- Thinly sliced carrots – ½ cup
- Julienned red pepper – ½ cup
- Fresh green beans – ½ cup
- Cooked white rice – 2 cups

Directions:

1. In a bowl, mix the lemon juice, garlic, ginger, and red pepper flakes.

2. Add the tofu and toss to coat.

3. Place the bowl in the refrigerator and marinate for 2 hours.

4. To make the stir-fry, heat the oil in a skillet.

5. Sauté the tofu for 8 minutes or until it is lightly browned and heated through.

6. Add the carrots, and cauliflower and sauté for 5 minutes. Stirring and tossing constantly.

7. Add the red pepper and green beans, sauté for 3 minutes more.

8. Serve over white rice.

Nutrition: Calories: 190 kcal; Total Fat: 6 g; Saturated Fat: 0 g; Cholesterol: 0 mg; Sodium: 22 mg; Total Carbs: 30 g; Fiber: 0 g; Sugar: 0 g; Protein: 6 g

# Chilaquiles

Preparation Time: 20 minutes

Cooking Time: 20 minutes

Servings: 4

Ingredients:

- 3 (8-inch) corn tortillas, cut into strips
- 2 tablespoons of extra-virgin olive oil
- 12 tomatillos, papery covering removed, chopped
- 3 tablespoons for freshly squeezed lime juice
- ⅛ teaspoon of salt
- ⅛ teaspoon of freshly ground black pepper
- 4 large egg whites
- 2 large eggs
- 2 tablespoons of water
- 1 cup of shredded pepper jack cheese

Directions:

1. In a dry nonstick skillet, toast the tortilla strips over medium heat until they are crisp, tossing the pan and stirring occasionally. This should take 4 to 6 minutes. Remove the strips from the pan and set aside.

2. In the same skillet, heat the olive oil over medium heat and add the tomatillos, lime juice, salt, and pepper. Cook and frequently stir for about 8 to 10 minutes until the tomatillos break down and form a sauce. Transfer the sauce to a bowl and set aside.

3.      In a small bowl, beat the egg whites, eggs, and water and add to the skillet. Cook the eggs for 3 to 4 minutes, stirring occasionally until they are set and cooked to 160°F.

4.      Preheat the oven to 400°F.

5.      Toss the tortilla strips in the tomatillo sauce and place in a casserole dish. Top with the scrambled eggs and cheese.

6.      Bake for 10 to 15 minutes, or until the cheese starts to brown. Serve.

Nutrition: Calories: 312 Total fat: 20g Saturated fat: 8g Sodium: 345mg Phosphorus: 280mg Potassium: 453mg Carbohydrates: 19g Fiber: 3g Protein: 15g Sugar: 5g

# Couscous Burgers

Preparation time: 20 minutes

Cooking time: 10 minutes

Servings: 4 servings

Ingredients:

- chickpeas – ½ cup
- Chopped fresh cilantro – 2 tbsp.
- Chopped fresh parsley
- Lemon juice - 1 tbsp.
- Lemon zest – 2 tsp
- Minced garlic – 1 tsp
- Cooked couscous – 2 ½ cups
- Eggs – 2, lightly beaten
- Olive oil – 2 tbsp.

Directions:

1. Put the cilantro, chickpeas, parsley, lemon juice, lemon zest, and garlic in a food processor and pulse until a paste form.

2. Transfer the chickpea mixture to a bowl, and add the eggs and couscous. Mix well.

3. Chill the mixture in the refrigerator for 1 hour.

4. Form the couscous mixture into 4 patties.

5. Heat olive oil in a skillet.

6. Place the patties in the skillet, 2 at a time, gently pressing them down with the fork of a spatula.

7.      Cook for 5 minutes or until golden, and flip the patties over.

8.      Cook the other side for 5 minutes and transfer the cooked burgers to a plate covered with a paper towel.

9.      Repeat with the remaining 2 burgers.

Nutrition: Calories: 242 kcal; Total Fat: 10 g; Saturated Fat: 0 g; Cholesterol: 0 mg; Sodium: 43 mg; Total Carbs: 29 g; Fiber: 0 g; Sugar: 0 g; Protein: 9 g

# Stir-Fried Gingery Veggies

Preparation Time: 10 minutes

Cooking Time: 10 minutes

Servings: 4

Ingredients:

- 1 tablespoon oil
- 3 cloves of garlic, minced
- 1 onion, chopped
- 1 thumb-size ginger, sliced
- 1 tablespoon water
- 1 large carrots, peeled and julienned and seedless
- 1 large green bell pepper, julienned and seedless
- 1 large yellow bell pepper, julienned and seedless
- 1 large red bell pepper, julienned and seedless
- 1 zucchini, julienned
- Salt and pepper to taste

Directions:

1.      Heat oil in a nonstick saucepan over a high flame and sauté the garlic, onion, and ginger until fragrant.

2.      Stir in the rest of the ingredients.

3.      Keep on stirring for at least 5 minutes until vegetables are tender.

4.      Serve and enjoy.

Nutrition: Calories 70 Total Fat 4g Saturated Fat 1g Total Carbs 9g Net Carbs 7g Protein 1g Sugar: 4g Fiber 2g Sodium 173mg Potassium 163mg

# Zucchini Bowl

Preparation Time: 10 minutes

Cooking Time: 20 minutes

Servings: 4

Ingredients:

- 1 onion, chopped
- 3 zucchini, cut into medium chunks
- 2 tablespoons coconut almond milk
- 2 garlic cloves, minced
- 4 cups chicken stock
- 2 tablespoons coconut oil
- Pinch of salt
- Black pepper to taste

Directions:

1. Take a pot and place it over medium heat
2. Add oil and let it heat up
3. Add zucchini, garlic, onion, and stir
4. Cook for 5 minutes
5. Add stock, salt, pepper, and stir
6. Bring to a boil and lower down the heat
7. Simmer for 20 minutes.
8. Remove heat and add coconut almond milk
9. Use an immersion blender until smooth
10. Ladle into soup bowls and serve

11.    Enjoy!

Nutrition: Calories: 160 Fat: 2g Carbohydrates: 4g Protein: 7g

# Fried Rice with Kale

Preparation Time: 10 minutes

Cooking Time: 12 minutes

Servings: 4

Ingredients:

- 2 tbsp. Extra virgin oil
- 8 oz. Tofu, chopped
- 6 Scallion, white and green parts, thinly sliced
- 2 cups Kale, stemmed and chopped
- 3 cups Cooked white rice
- ¼ cup Stir fry sauce

Directions:

1. In a huge skillet on medium-high heat, warm the oil until it shimmers.

2. Add the tofu, scallions, and kale. Cook for 5 to 7 minutes, frequently stirring, until the vegetables are soft.

3. Add the white rice and stir-fry sauce. Cook for 3 to 5 minutes, occasionally stirring, until heated through.

Nutrition: Calories: 301 Total Fat: 11g Total Carbs: 36g Sugar: 1g Fiber: 3g Protein: 16g  Sodium: 2,535mg

# Curried Veggie Stir-Fry

Preparation Time: 20 minutes

Cooking Time: 10 minutes

Servings: 6

Ingredients:

- 2 tablespoons of extra-virgin olive oil
- 1 onion, chopped
- 4 garlic cloves, minced
- 4 cups of frozen stir-fry vegetables
- 1 cup unsweetened full-fat coconut almond milk
- 1 cup of water
- 2 tablespoons of green curry paste

Directions:

1. In a wok or non-stick, heat the olive oil over medium-high heat. Stir-fry the onion and garlic for 2 to 3 minutes, until fragrant.

2. Add the frozen stir-fry vegetables and continue to cook for 3 to 4 minutes longer, or until the vegetables are hot.

3. Meanwhile, in a small bowl, combine coconut almond milk, water, and curry paste. Stir until the paste dissolves.

4. Add the broth mixture to the wok and cook for another 2 to 3 minutes, or until the sauce has reduced slightly and all the vegetables are crisp-tender.

5. Serve over couscous or hot cooked rice.

Nutrition: Calories: 293 Total fat: 18g Saturated fat: 10g Sodium: 247mg Phosphorus: 138mg Potassium: 531mg Carbohydrates: 28g Fiber: 7g Protein: 7g Sugar: 4g

# Nice Coconut Haddock

Preparation Time: 10 minutes

Cooking Time: 12 minutes

Servings: 3

Ingredients:

- 4 haddock fillets, 5 ounces each, boneless
- 2 tablespoons coconut oil, melted
- 1 cup coconut, shredded and unsweetened
- ¼ cup hazelnuts, ground
- Salt to taste

Directions:

1. Preheat your oven to 400 °F
2. Line a baking sheet with parchment paper
3. Keep it on the side
4. Pat fish fillets with a paper towel and season with salt
5. Take a bowl and stir in hazelnuts and shredded coconut
6. Drag fish fillets through the coconut mix until both sides are coated well
7. Transfer to a baking dish
8. Brush with coconut oil
9. Bake for about 12 minutes until flaky
10. Serve and enjoy!

Nutrition: Calories: 299 Fat: 24g Carbohydrates: 1g Protein: 20g

# Lime Green lettuce and Chickpeas Salad

Preparation Time: 10 minutes

Cooking Time: 0 minutes

Servings: 4

Ingredients:

- 16 ounces canned chickpeas, drained and rinsed
- 2 cups baby green lettuce leaves
- ½ tablespoon lime juice
- 2 tablespoons olive oil
- 1 teaspoon cumin, ground
- Sea salt and black pepper
- ½ teaspoon chili flakes

Directions:

1.     In a bowl, mix the chickpeas with the green lettuce and the rest of the ingredients, toss and serve cold.

Nutrition: Calories 240, Fat 8.2, Fiber 5.3, Carbs 11.6, Protein 12

# Dinner

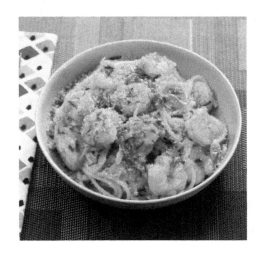

# Ground Turkey with Peas & Potato

Preparation Time: 15 minutes

Cooking Time: 35 minutes

Servings: 4

Ingredients:

- 3-4 tablespoons coconut oil
- 1-pound lean ground turkey
- 1-2 fresh red chilis, chopped
- 1 onion, chopped
- Salt, to taste
- 2 minced garlic cloves
- 1 (1-inch) piece fresh ginger, grated finely
- 1 tablespoon curry powder
- 1 teaspoon ground coriander
- 1 teaspoon ground cumin
- 1 teaspoon ground turmeric
- 2 large Yukon gold carrots, cubed into 1-inch size
- ½ cup of water
- 1 cup fresh peas, shelled
- 2-4 plum Red bell peppers, chopped
- ½ cup fresh cilantro, chopped

Directions:

1. In a substantial pan, heat oil on medium-high heat. Add turkey and cook for about 4-5 minutes. Add chilis and onion and cook for about 4-5 minutes.

2.     Add garlic and ginger and cook approximately 1-2 minutes. Stir in spices, carrots, and water and convey to your boil

3.     Reduce the warmth to medium-low. Simmer covered around 15-20 or so minutes. Add peas and Red bell peppers and cook for about 2-3 minutes. Serve using the garnishing of cilantro.

Nutrition: Calories: 452 Fat: 14g Carbohydrates: 24g Fiber: 13g Protein: 36g Phosphorus 38 mg Potassium 99.5 mg Sodium 373.4 mg

# Turkey & Pumpkin Chili

Preparation Time: 15 minutes

Cooking Time: 41 minutes

Servings: 4-6

Ingredients:

- 2 tablespoons extra-virgin olive oil
- 1 green bell pepper, seeded and chopped
- 1 small yellow onion, chopped
- 2 garlic cloves, chopped finely
- 1-pound lean ground turkey
- 1 (15-ounce) pumpkin puree
- 1 (14 ½-ounce) can diced Red bell peppers with liquid
- 1 teaspoon ground cumin
- ½ teaspoon ground turmeric
- ½ teaspoon ground cinnamon
- 1 cup of water
- 1 can chickpeas, rinsed and drained

Directions:

1. Heat-up oil on medium-low heat in a big pan. Add the bell pepper, onion, and garlic and sauté for approximately 5 minutes. Add turkey and cook for about 5-6 minutes.

2. Add Red bell peppers, pumpkin, spices, and water and convey to your boil on high heat. Reduce the temperature to medium-low heat and stir in chickpeas. Simmer, covered for approximately a half-hour, stirring occasionally. Serve hot.

Nutrition: Calories: 437 Fat: 17g Carbohydrates: 29g Protein: 42g Phosphorus 150 mg Potassium 652 mg Sodium 570 mg

# Ground Turkey with Asparagus

Preparation Time: 15 minutes

Cooking Time: 15 minutes

Servings: 8

Ingredients:

- 1¾ pound lean ground turkey
- 2 tablespoons sesame oil
- 1 medium onion, chopped
- 1 cup celery, chopped
- 6 garlic cloves, minced
- 2 cups asparagus, cut into 1-inch pieces
- 1/3 cup coconut aminos
- 2½ teaspoons ginger powder
- 2 tablespoons organic coconut crystals
- 1 tablespoon arrowroot starch
- 1 tablespoon cold water
- ¼ teaspoon red pepper flakes, crushed

Directions:

1. Heat a substantial nonstick skillet on medium-high heat. Add turkey and cook for approximately 5-7 minutes or till browned. With a slotted spoon, transfer the turkey inside a bowl and discard the grease from the skillet.

2. Heat-up oil on medium heat in the same skillet. Add onion, celery, and garlic and sauté for about 5 minutes. Add asparagus and cooked turkey, minimizing the temperature to medium-low.

3.      Meanwhile, inside a pan, mix coconut aminos, ginger powder, and coconut crystals n medium heat and convey some boil.

4.      Mix arrowroot starch and water in a smaller bowl. Slowly add arrowroot mixture, stirring continuously. Cook approximately 2-3 minutes.

5.      Add the sauce in the skillet with turkey mixture and stir to blend. Stir in red pepper flakes and cook for approximately 2-3 minutes. Serve hot.

Nutrition: Calories: 309 Fat: 20g Carbohydrates: 19g Protein: 28g Potassium 196.4 mg Sodium 77.8 mg Phosphorus 0 mg

# Chicken curry

Preparation Time: 10 minutes

Cooking Time: 4 minutes

Servings: 4

Ingredients

- 1lb skinless chicken breasts
- 1 medium onion, thinly sliced
- 1 15 ounce can chickpeas, drained and rinsed well
- ½ cup light coconut almond milk
- ½ cup chicken stock (see recipe)
- 1 15ounce can sodium-free tomato sauce
- 2 tablespoon curry powder
- 1 teaspoon low-sodium salt
- ½ cayenne powder
- 1 cup green peas
- 2 tablespoon lemon juice

Directions

1. Place the chicken breasts, onion, chickpeas into a 4 to 6-quart slow cooker.

2. Mix the coconut almond milk, chicken stock, tomato sauce, curry powder, salt, and cayenne together and pour into the slow cooker, stirring to coat well.

3. Cover and cook on low for 8 hours or high for 4 hours.

4. Stir in the peas and lemon juice 5 minutes before serving.

Nutrition: calories 302, fat 5g, carbs 43g, protein 24g, fiber 9g, potassium 573mg, sodium 800mg

# Poultry

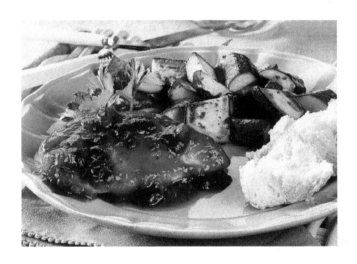

# Chicken Veronique

Preparation Time: 10 minutes

Cooking Time: 10 minutes

Servings: 4

Ingredients:

- 2 boneless skinless chicken breasts
- 1/2 shallot, chopped
- 2 tablespoons butter
- 2 tablespoons dry white wine
- 2 tablespoons chicken broth
- 1/2 cup green grapes, halved
- 1 teaspoon dried tarragon
- 1/4 cup cream

Directions:

1. Place an 8-inch skillet over medium heat and add butter to melt.

2. Sear the chicken in the melted butter until golden-brown on both sides.

3. Place the boneless chicken on a plate and set it aside.

4. Add shallot to the same skillet and stir until soft.

5. Whisk cornstarch with broth and wine in a small bowl.

6. Pour this slurry into the skillet and mix well.

7. Place the chicken in the skillet and cook it on a simmer for 6 minutes.

8. Transfer the chicken to the serving plate.

9. Add cream, tarragon, and grapes.

10.    Cook for 1 minute, and then pour this sauce over the chicken.

11.    Serve.

Nutrition: Calories: 306 kcal Total Fat: 18 g Saturated Fat: 0 g Cholesterol: 124 mg Sodium: 167 mg Total Carbs: 9 g

# Creamy Parsnip Soup

Preparation Time: 25 minutes

Cooking Time: 60 minutes

Servings: 10

Ingredients:

- 2 pounds parsnips (peeled, cut)
- 3 carrots (peeled, cut)
- 4 cups chicken stock
- 1 large onion (diced)
- 3 stalks celery (diced)
- 3 cloves garlic (minced)
- 1 teaspoon ground ginger
- 1/2 teaspoon ground cardamom
- 1/2 teaspoon ground allspice
- 1/2 teaspoon ground nutmeg
- 1/4 teaspoon cayenne pepper
- 1 tablespoon brown sugar
- 1 cup whole almond milk
- 1 tablespoon butter
- 1 tablespoon olive oil
- Salt
- Ground black pepper

Directions:

1. Preheat oven to 425 F.

2. Toss the parsnips and carrots with oil and seasoning in a bowl. Place them over a baking sheet.

3.     Roast in oven until for 30 minutes.

4.     Cook the onion and celery in oil till golden brown, about 7 minutes. Add butter, brown sugar, garlic, and the parsnips and carrots, cooking for 10 minutes.

5.     Season and stir. Add the chicken stock to a boil until tender.

6.     Puree the soup.

7.     Add almond milk and cream and simmer some more before serving with seasoning.

Nutrition: Calories: 187 kcal Carbs: 24 g Fat: 9 g Protein: 3 g

# London Broil

Preparation Time: 10 minutes

Cooking Time: 5 minutes

Servings: 4

Ingredients:

- 2 pounds flank steak
- 1/4 teaspoon meat tenderizer
- 1 tablespoon sugar
- 2 tablespoons lemon juice
- 2 tablespoons soy sauce
- 1 tablespoon honey
- 1 teaspoon herb seasoning blend

Directions:

1. Pound the meat with a mallet then place it in a shallow dish.

2. Sprinkle meat tenderizer over the meat.

3. Whisk rest of the ingredients and spread this marinade over the meat.

4. Marinate the meat for 4 hours in the refrigerator.

5. Bake the meat for 5 minutes per side at 350°F.

6. Slice and serve.

Nutrition: Calories: 184 kcal Total Fat: 8 g Saturated Fat: 0 g Cholesterol: 43 mg Sodium: 208 mg Total Carbs: 3 g

# Butternut Squash Soup with Shrimp

Preparation Time: 10 minutes

Cooking Time: 20 minutes

Servings: 4

Ingredients:

- 3 tablespoons unsalted butter
- 1 small red onion, finely chopped
- 1 garlic clove, sliced
- 1 teaspoon turmeric
- 1 teaspoon salt
- ¼ teaspoon freshly ground black pepper
- 3 cups vegetable broth
- 2 cups peeled butternut squash cut into ¼-inch dice
- 1 pound cooked peeled shrimp, thawed if necessary
- 1 cup unsweetened almond milk
- ¼ cup slivered almonds (optional)
- 2 tablespoons finely chopped fresh flat-leaf parsley
- 2 teaspoons grated or minced lemon zest

Directions:

1. In a huge pot, melt the butter on high heat.

2. Add the onion, garlic, turmeric, salt, and pepper and sauté until the vegetables are soft and translucent, 5 to 7 minutes.

3. Add the broth and squash and bring to a boil.

4. Lower the heat and cook until the squash has softened, about 5 minutes.

5.  Add the shrimp and almond milk and cook until heated through, about 2 minutes.

6.  Sprinkle with the almonds (if using), parsley, and lemon zest and serve.

Nutrition: Calories: 275 Total Fat: 12g Total Carbohydrates: 12g Sugar: 3g Fiber: 2g; Protein: 30g Sodium: 1665mg

# Chicken and Apple Curry

Preparation Time: 10 minutes

Cooking Time: 1 hour and 11 minutes

Servings: 8

Ingredients:

- 8 boneless skinless chicken breasts
- 1/4 teaspoon black pepper
- 2 medium apples, peeled, cored, and chopped
- 2 small onions, chopped
- 1 garlic clove, minced
- 3 tablespoons butter
- 1 tablespoon curry powder
- 1/2 tablespoon dried basil
- 3 tablespoons flour
- 1 cup chicken broth
- 1 cup of rice almond milk

Directions:

1. Preheat oven to 350°F.

2. Set the chicken breasts in a baking pan and sprinkle black pepper over it.

3. Place a suitably-sized saucepan over medium heat and add butter to melt.

4. Add onion, garlic, and apple, then sauté until soft.

5. Stir in basil and curry powder, and then cook for 1 minute.

6. Add flour and continue mixing for 1 minute.

7. Stir in rice almond milk and chicken broth, then stir cook for 5 minutes.

8. Pour this sauce over the chicken breasts in the baking pan.

9. Bake the chicken for 60 minutes then serve.

Nutrition: Calories: 232 kcal Total Fat: 8 g Saturated Fat: 0 g Cholesterol: 85 mg Sodium: 118 mg Total Carbs: 11 g

# Clear Clam Chowder

Preparation Time: 10 minutes

Cooking Time: 15 minutes

Servings: 4

Ingredients:

- 2 tablespoons unsalted butter
- 2 medium carrots, cut into ½-inch pieces
- 2 celery stalks, thinly sliced
- 1 small red onion, cut into ¼-inch dice
- 2 garlic cloves, sliced
- 2 cups vegetable broth
- 1 (8-ounce) bottle clam juice
- 1 (10-ounce) can clams
- ½ teaspoon dried thyme
- ½ teaspoon salt
- ¼ teaspoon freshly ground black pepper

Directions:

1.    In a huge pot, melt the butter on high heat.

2.    Add the carrots, celery, onion, and garlic and sauté until slightly softened 2 to 3 minutes.

3.    Pour the broth and clam juice, then bring it to a boil.

4.    Lower the heat and cook until the carrots are soft, 3 to 5 minutes.

5.     Stir in the clams and their juices, thyme, salt, and pepper, heat through for 2 to 3 minutes, and serve.

Nutrition: Calories: 156 Total Fat: 7g Total Carbohydrates: 7g Sugar: 3g Fiber: 1g Protein: 14g Sodium: 981mg

# Cream of Mushroom Soup

Preparation Time: 20 minutes

Cooking Time: 30 minutes

Servings: 6

Ingredients:

- 5 cups mushrooms (sliced)
- 1-1/2 cups chicken broth
- 1 tablespoon sherry
- 3 tablespoons butter
- 3 tablespoons flour
- 1 cup half-and-half
- 1/8 teaspoon dried thyme
- 1/2 cup onion (chopped)
- Salt
- Ground black pepper

Directions:

1.	Cook mushrooms with onion and thyme in the broth until tender.

2.	Puree the mixture.

3.      Whisk some flour in a pan of melted butter. Add half-and-half, vegetable puree, and seasoning. Boil until thickened.

4.      Add sherry.

Nutrition: Calories: 148 kcal Carbs: 8.6 g Fat: 11 g Protein: 4 g

# Saffron and Salmon Soup

Preparation Time: 10 minutes

Cooking Time: 20 minutes

Servings: 4

Ingredients:

- ¼ cup extra-virgin olive oil
- 2 leeks, white parts only, thinly sliced
- 2 medium carrots, thinly sliced
- 2 garlic cloves, thinly sliced
- 4 cups vegetable broth
- 1 lb. salmon fillets, cut into 1-inch pieces
- 1 tsp. salt
- ¼ tsp. freshly ground black pepper
- ¼ tsp. saffron threads
- 2 cups baby spinach
- ½ cup dry white wine
- 2 tablespoons chopped scallions, both white and green parts
- 2 tablespoons finely chopped fresh flat-leaf parsley

Directions:

1. In a huge pot, heat the oil over high heat.

2. Add the leeks, carrots, and garlic and sauté until softened, 5 to 7 minutes.

3. Pour the broth then bring to a boil.

4.    Lower the heat to a simmer then add the salmon, salt, pepper, and saffron. Cook until the salmon is cooked through, at least 8 minutes.

5.    Add the spinach, wine, scallions, and parsley and cook until the spinach has wilted, 1 to 2 minutes, and serve.

Nutrition: Calories: 418 Total Fat: 26g Total Carbohydrates: 13g Sugar: 4g Fiber: 2g Protein: 29g Sodium: 1455mg

# Cannellini Bean Soup

Preparation Time: 25 minutes

Cooking Time: 30 minutes

Servings: 6

Ingredients:

- 2 slices smoked bacon (chopped)
- 6 cups chicken broth
- 1 cannellini beans
- 1 bunch red Swiss chard
- 2 tablespoons chopped sun-dried bell pepper
- 2 ounces Parmesan cheese rind
- 1 onion (chopped)
- 1 clove garlic (minced)
- 5 large sage leaves (minced)
- 5 leaves basil (chopped)
- 1/4 teaspoon nutmeg (grated)
- 1/8 teaspoon red pepper flakes (crushed)
- 1 tablespoon extra-virgin olive oil

Directions:

1. Cook the bacon with garlic, onion, nutmeg, and red pepper flakes for 5 minutes.

2. Pour in beans, chicken broth, sun-dried bell pepper, and Parmesan cheese rind, simmering for 10 minutes.

3. Add the cut chard and chard leaves into the soup.

4. Simmer and then add into bowls with a drizzle of oil and Parmesan cheese.

Nutrition: Calories: 215 kcal Carbs: 23 g Fat: 10 g Protein: 9.7 g

# Snack

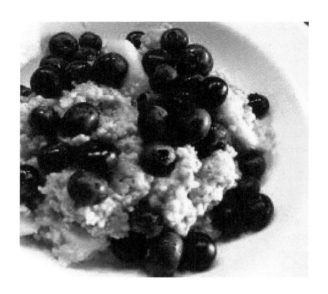

# Fragrant Thai-Style Eggplant

Preparation Time: 10 minutes

Cooking Time: 20 minutes

Serving: 6

Ingredients:

- 1 eggplant, cut into ½-inch slices
- ¼ teaspoon salt
- 1 tablespoon extra-virgin olive oil
- 1 tablespoon peeled and grated fresh ginger root
- 1 garlic clove, minced
- 2 tablespoons freshly squeezed lime juice
- 1 tablespoon water
- 2 tablespoons chopped fresh basil

Direction

1. Preheat the oven to 400°F.

2. On a baking sheet with a lip, arrange the eggplant slices and sprinkle evenly with the salt. Drizzle with the olive oil.

3. Bake the eggplant for 10 minutes, then remove the baking sheet from the oven and turn the slices over. Return the baking sheet to the oven and bake for 10 to 15 minutes longer or until the eggplant is tender.

4. Meanwhile, stir together the ginger, garlic, lime juice, water, and basil in a small bowl until well mixed.

5. Situate the eggplant on a serving plate and drizzle with the ginger mixture. Serve warm or cool.

Nutrition: 52 Calories 101mg Sodium 30mg Phosphorus 280mg Potassium 1g Protein

# Roasted Asparagus with Pine Nuts

Preparation Time: 10 minutes

Cooking Time: 13 minutes

Serving: 4

Ingredients:

- 1-pound fresh asparagus, woody ends removed
- 1 tablespoon olive oil
- 1 tablespoon balsamic vinegar
- 3 garlic cloves, minced
- ½ teaspoon dried thyme leaves
- ¼ cup pine nuts

Direction

1. Preheat the oven to 400°F.

2. Rinse the asparagus and arrange in a single layer on a baking sheet.

3. Blend olive oil, balsamic vinegar, garlic, and thyme until well mixed.

4. Drizzle the dressing over the asparagus and toss to coat.

5. Roast the asparagus for 10 minutes and remove the baking sheet from the oven.

6. Sprinkle the pine nuts over the asparagus and return the baking sheet to the oven. Roast for another 5 to 7 minutes or until the pine nuts are toasted and the asparagus is tender and light golden brown. Serve.

Nutrition: 116 Calories 4mg Sodium 112mg Phosphorus 294mg Potassium 4g Protein

# Roasted Radishes

Preparation Time: 10 minutes

Cooking Time: 20 minutes

Serving: 6

Ingredients:

- 3 bunches whole small radishes
- 3 tablespoons olive oil, divided
- 1 tablespoon freshly squeezed lemon juice
- 1 tablespoon Dijon mustard
- ½ teaspoon dried marjoram leaves
- 1/8 teaspoon white pepper
- Pinch salt
- 2 tablespoons chopped flat-leaf parsley

Direction

1. Preheat the oven to 425°F. Prep a baking sheet with a lip with parchment paper and set aside.

2. Scrub the radishes, remove the stem and root, and cut each in half or thirds, depending on the size. The radishes should be similarly sized, so they cook evenly.

3. Toss the radishes and 1 tablespoon olive oil on the baking sheet to coat and arrange the radishes in a single layer.

4. Roast the radishes for 18 to 20 minutes or until they are slightly golden and tender, but still crisp on the outside.

5.      While the radishes are roasting, whisk together the remaining 2 tablespoons of olive oil with the lemon juice, mustard, marjoram, pepper, and salt in a small bowl.

6.      Once done, take them from the baking sheet and place them in a serving bowl. Drizzle the vegetables with the dressing and toss. Sprinkle with the parsley. Serve warm or cool.

Nutrition: 79 Calories 123mg Sodium 23mg Phosphorus 232mg Potassium 1g Protein

# Sautéed Spicy Cabbage

Preparation Time: 15 minutes

Cooking Time: 5 minutes

Serving: 6

Ingredients:

- 3 tablespoons olive oil
- 3 cups chopped green cabbage
- 3 cups chopped red cabbage
- 2 garlic cloves, minced
- 1/8 teaspoon cayenne pepper
- Pinch salt

Direction

1. Cook olive oil in a large skillet over medium heat.

2. Stir in red and green cabbage and the garlic; sauté until the leaves wilt and are tender, about 4 to 5 minutes.

3. Sprinkle the vegetables with the cayenne pepper and salt, toss, and serve.

Nutrition: 86 Calories 46mg Sodium 27mg Phosphorus 189mg Potassium 1g Protein

# Herbed Garlic Cauliflower Mash

Preparation Time: 10 minutes

Cooking Time: 20 minutes

Serving: 6

Ingredients:

- 4 cups cauliflower florets
- 4 garlic cloves, peeled
- 4 ounces cream cheese, softened
- ¼ cup unsweetened almond almond milk
- 2 tablespoons unsalted butter
- Pinch salt
- 2 tablespoons minced fresh chives
- 2 tablespoons chopped flat-leaf parsley
- 1 tablespoon fresh thyme leaves

Direction

1.      Boil water at high heat. Add the cauliflower and garlic and cook, stirring occasionally, until the cauliflower is tender, about 8 to 10 minutes.

2.      Drain the cauliflower and garlic into a colander in the sink and shake the colander well to remove excess water.

3.      Using a paper towel, blot the vegetables to remove any remaining water. Return the florets to the pot and place over low heat for 1 minute to remove as much water as possible.

4.      Mash the florets and garlic with a potato masher until smooth.

5.      Beat in the cream cheese, almond almond milk, butter, salt, chives, parsley, and thyme with a spoon. Serve.

Nutrition: 124 Calories 115mg Sodium 59mg Phosphorus 266mg Potassium 3g Protein

# Desserts

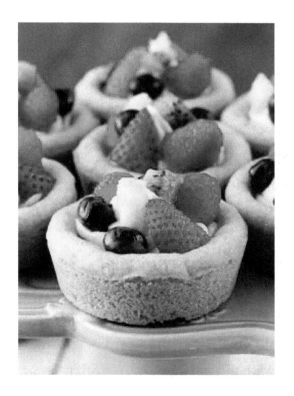

# Gumdrop Cookies

Preparation Time: 15 minutes

Cooking Time: 12 minutes

Servings: 25

Ingredients:

- ½ cup of spreadable unsalted butter
- 1 medium egg
- 1 cup of brown sugar
- 1 ⅔ cups of all-purpose flour, sifted
- ¼ cup of almond milk
- 1 teaspoon vanilla
- 1 teaspoon of baking powder
- 15 large gumdrops, chopped finely

Directions:

1. Preheat the oven at 400F/195C.

2. Combine the sugar, butter and egg until creamy.

3. Add the almond milk and vanilla and stir well.

4. Combine the flour with the baking powder in a different bowl. Incorporate to the sugar, butter mixture, and stir.

5. Add the gumdrops and place the mixture in the fridge for half an hour.

6. Drop the dough with tablespoonful into a lightly greased baking or cookie sheet.

7. Bake for 10-12 minutes or until golden brown.

Nutrition: Calories: 102.17 kcal Carbohydrate: 16.5 g Protein: 0.86 g Sodium: 23.42 mg Potassium: 45 mg Phosphorus: 32.15 mg Dietary Fiber: 0.13 g Fat: 4 g

# Old-fashioned Apple Kuchen

Preparation time: 25 minutes

Cook time: 1 hour

Servings: 16

Ingredients:

- Unsalted butter, for greasing the baking dish
- 1 cup unsalted butter, at room temperature
- 2 cups granulated sugar
- 2 eggs, beaten
- 2 teaspoons pure vanilla extract
- 2 cups all-purpose flour
- 1 teaspoon Ener-G baking soda substitute
- 2 teaspoons ground cinnamon
- ½ teaspoon ground nutmeg
- Pinch ground allspice
- 2 large apples, peeled, cored, and diced (about 3 cups)

Directions:

1. Preheat the oven to 350°F.

2. Grease a 9-by-13-inch glass baking dish; set aside.

3. Cream together the butter and sugar with a hand mixer until light and fluffy, for about 3 minutes.

4. Add the eggs and vanilla and beat until combined, scraping down the sides of the bowl, about 1 minute.

5. In a small bowl, stir together the flour, baking soda substitute, cinnamon, nutmeg, and allspice.

6.     Add the dry ingredients to the wet ingredients and stir to combine.

7.     Stir in the apple and spoon the batter into the baking dish.

8.     Bake for about 1 hour or until the cake is golden.

9.     Cool the cake on a wire rack.

10.     Serve warm or chilled.

Nutrition: Calories: 368; Fat: 16g; Carbohydrates: 53g; Phosphorus: 46mg; Potassium: 68mg; Sodium: 15mg; Protein: 3g

# Dessert Cocktail

Preparation Time: 1 minutes

Cooking Time: 0 minute

Servings: 4

Ingredients:

- 1 cup of cranberry juice
- 1 cup of fresh ripe strawberries, washed and hull removed
- 2 tablespoon of lime juice
- ¼ cup of white sugar
- 8 ice cubes

Directions:

1. Combine all the ingredients in a blender until smooth and creamy.

2. Pour the liquid into chilled tall glasses and serve cold.

Nutrition: Calories: 92 kcal Carbohydrate: 23.5 g Protein: 0.5 g Sodium: 3.62 mg Potassium: 103.78 mg Phosphorus: 17.86 mg Dietary Fiber: 0.84 g Fat: 0.17 g

# Baked Egg Custard

Preparation Time: 15 minutes

Cooking Time: 30 minutes

Servings: 4

Ingredients:

- 2 medium eggs, at room temperature
- ¼ cup of semi-skimmed almond milk
- 3 tablespoons of white sugar
- ½ teaspoon of nutmeg
- 1 teaspoon of vanilla extract

Directions:

1. Preheat your oven at 375 F/180C
2. Mix all the ingredients in a mixing bowl and beat with a hand mixer for a few seconds until creamy and uniform.
3. Pour the mixture into lightly greased muffin tins.
4. Bake for 25-30 minutes or until the knife, you place inside, comes out clean.

Nutrition: Calories: 96.56 kcal Carbohydrate: 10.5 g Protein: 3.5 g Sodium: 37.75 mg Potassium: 58.19 mg Phosphorus: 58.76 mg

Dietary Fiber: 0.06 g Fat: 2.91 g

CPSIA information can be obtained
at www.ICGtesting.com
Printed in the USA
LVHW051100010621
689026LV00008B/1125